CONTENTS

CHAPTER 4

CHAPTER 5

CHAPTER 6

CHAPTER 7

INTRODUCTION

It might surprise you to learn that one of the most common health problems in this country today is also one of the easiest to correct. Hypoglycemia or low blood sugar has been estimated to effect anywhere from 50 million to 150 million people in this country alone.

Hypoglycemia has never received enormous amounts of publicity like cancer, AIDS or diabetes, but that's not because it's only a minor inconvenience compared to these diseases. In fact, hypoglycemia is now suspected to be the "hidden force" contributing to the over-crowding in our prisons and mental institutions, increased alcoholism, divorce rate and child abuse. Even our nations third largest killer,diabetes,can stem from uncorrected hypoglycemia.

If low blood sugar is such a problem, why hasn't everyone been informed? New,life-threatening diseases like AIDS,have triggered massive publicity campaigns. Complete multi-million dollar corporate organizations have evolved to provide information about cancer, heart disease, diabetes, cystic fibrosis, M.S. and a host of other, even less threatening diseases that effect far less people than hypoglycemia. So it seems reasonable if hypoglycemia was such a big problem, we'd hear more about it. Right?

Let's face it, hypoglycemia is not a popular condition. For one thing, there's no money to be made in treating the problem. It can be completely eliminated with changes in the diet (certain nutritional supplements can help speed up the corrective process). It's just not the type of condition that needs the discovery of a new miracle drug. Expensive long-term research studies aren't necessary to discover its cause - we already know it. Even if some well-meaning corporation or organization embarked on a hypoglycemia awareness campaign, there would be no way to recoup expenses. In short, treating hypoglycemia is not profitable. But on the other hand, ignoring low blood sugar problems can generate billions of dollars!

The fast food, soft drink, candy, alcoholic beverage industries and the majority of over-the-counter pharmaceutical manufacturers knowingly or unknowingly are to a very large degree dependent on the hypoglycemics in this country.

Mass advertising on TV and in magazines refer to the symptoms of hypoglycemia as normal, everyday, acceptable events. Everyone has a ready answer for those "everyday headaches, fatigue, joint and muscle aches, insomnia, hunger pains and nervousness." Everything from drugs to candy bars are offered to help us cope with the problems of a stressful lifestyle.

Our society has a long way to go in even recognizing that a hypoglycemia problem exists. Even though the problem was first recognized over 60 years ago, it is still difficult to find physicians who have a thorough understanding of the problem. Unfortunately, I don't think we're going to see any drastic changes in the way hypoglycemia problems are addressed in this country. Basically, you're on your own when it comes to dealing with a low blood sugar problem.

Before we go into more specifics about low blood sugar, just for fun, grab a pencil and answer the questions on the following pages. They will only take a minute or so and you shouldn't have any problem deciding on the correct answers. They are simple questions, unless you just finished a cup of coffee with sugar and a sweet roll. (Low blood sugar does cause indecisiveness and confusion.)

CHAPTER 1

LOW BLOOD SUGAR EVALUATION

Just to see how you stand regarding hypoglycemia (low blood sugar) read each of the following short questions and answer each by circling either yes or no.

1. Do you skip breakfast in the mornings?
   Yes No

2. Do you feel hungry shortly after eating?
   Yes No

3. Do you often skip meals?
   Yes No

4. Do you wake sometimes during the night feeling hungry?
   Yes No

5. Do you wake up during the night and have a hard time getting back to sleep?
   Yes No

6. Do your feet and hands seem to get cold often?

Yes No

7. Do you ever feel knotting or cramping in the stomach?

Yes No

8. Do you get dizzy when you stand up quickly?

Yes No

9. Do you sometimes become irritable or shaky if you skip a meal?

Yes No

10. Have you ever had a nervous breakdown?

Yes No

11. Do you feel better after you eat?

Yes No

12. Do you occasionally have a rapid heart beat for no apparent reason?

Yes No

13. Does it seem like you're always hungry?

Yes No

14. Do you have occasional numbness in your legs and arms?

Yes No

15. When you walk outside does bright sunlight bother your eyes?

Yes No

16. Do you get a headache if you go too long without eating?

Yes No

17. Do you feel nervous frequently?
Yes No

18. Do you have leg cramps?
Yes No

19. Do you have nightmares?
Yes No

20. Do you still feel tired even after sleeping through the night?
Yes No

21. Do you ever cry for no reason at all?
Yes No

22. Do you ever feel like you`re in a daze (out of touch with reality)?
Yes No

23. Do you often find it hard to concentrate?
Yes No

24. Do you have cravings for sweets, chocolate or alcoholic beverages?
Yes No

25. Do you have pain in your joints?
Yes No

26. Have you ever thought of committing suicide?
Yes No

27. Are you frequently depressed?
Yes No

28. Are you irritable first thing in the morning before breakfast or your first cup of coffee?
Yes No

29. Do you ever have cold clammy sweats?
Yes No

30. Do you experience twitching or jerking of muscles?
Yes No

31. Does your vision ever become blurred for no reason?
Yes No

32. Do you get weak or shaky if you skip a meal?
Yes No

33. Do you find it difficult to make a decision?
Yes No

34. Have you experienced a drop in sex drive?
Yes No

35. Do you snack on sweets between meals?
Yes No

36. Do you get headaches behind your eyes?
Yes No

37. Are you overweight from the waist down?
Yes No

38. Do you sometimes have swelling (water retention) in the ankles, feet or fingers?
Yes No

39. Do you frequently feel drowsy?
Yes No

40. Do you ever experience shortness of breath?
Yes No

41. Do you have a hard time remembering things?
Yes No

42. Do you sometimes feel uncoordinated?
Yes No

43. Do you ever have smothering spells?
Yes No

44. Do you have problems with asthma?
Yes No

45. Are you overweight from the waist up?
Yes No

46. Do you drink more than 3 cups of coffee a day?
Yes No

47. Do you drink one or more soft drinks a day?
Yes No

48. Do you smoke?
Yes No

49. Do you find it more difficult to concentrate in the afternoon?
Yes No

50. Have you ever blacked out?
Yes No

51. Do you have allergy problems?
Yes No

52. Do you have more energy at night than you do in the daytime?

Yes No

53. Do you eat chocolate or candy over three times a week?

Yes No

54. Has anyone in your family had diabetes?

Yes No

55. Do you oftentimes have unrealistic fears?

Yes No

56. Do you experience hangovers when you drink alcohol?

Yes No

57. Do you have night sweats?

Yes No

58. Do you seem to sigh and yawn frequently?

Yes No

59. Do you have to urinate frequently?

Yes No

60. Does alcohol go to your head quickly?

Yes No

61. Would you like to know what the answers to the questions have to do with low blood sugar? Then count the number of questions you answered yes to and turn the page.

If you answered 20 or more of the questions with "yes", there's a very strong possibility you have problems with hypoglycemia. Less than 20, you may not, but if you're sipping on a soft drink or cup of coffee or feel like you need a snack after that tough test......keep on reading!

Seriously, if you had over 20 "yes" answers, you are going to find this book especially interesting. In fact, at times, you'll probably think it was written specifically about you. You'll be surprised to learn just how many health problems can now be linked directly to low blood sugar. Even more surprising will be how simply the problems can be eliminated!

Let's take a closer look at what causes hypoglycemia and why the symptoms associated with it are so predictable.

CHAPTER 2

WHAT IS HYPOGLYCEMIA (Low Blood Sugar)?

Hypoglycemia is not a disease. It's not some type of infection nor is it caused by some mysterious virus. Hypoglycemia is simply low blood sugar. ("Hypo" placed before any word means under or below. Glycemia means sugar in the blood. Hypoglycemia = low blood sugar).

Hypoglycemia was discovered by Dr. Seale Harris in 1924. Twenty-five years later, he was awarded the Distinguished Service Medal from the American Medical Association (AMA) for his discovery. It has now been over sixty years since his discovery and hypoglycemia continues to be a growing epidemic with no end in sight. In 1957, Dr. S.P. Gyland made the following statement in an address to the AMA. "There is probably no illness today which causes such widespread suffering, so much inefficiency and loss of time, so many accidents, so many family breakups, and so many suicides as that of hypoglycemia." This same statement still rings true today...over thirty years later!

When we talk about blood sugar; we're really talking about glucose. Glucose is your main source of energy. It's the fuel that makes your body run. Your brain needs glucose to make decisions and solve problems, muscles need it for strength; in fact, you are dependant on glucose to stay alive. The glucose levels in your blood are a very serious matter and just to maintain the proper levels requires the coordinated efforts of several major organs.

To best explain how your body regulates blood sugar levels, let's look at what happens when you eat a meal.

"NO PROBLEM"

As digestion takes place, foods are changed into glucose. Glucose (sugar) levels in the bloodstream begin to rise. This triggers the pancreas to secrete insulin which helps pull glucose out of the blood and carry it into cells where it can either be used for energy or stored for later use. As the glucose level falls, the adrenal glands are triggered to release a hormone called cortisol. Cortisol in effect helps neutralize insulin and also helps release extra glucose that has been stored in the liver. If everything works as normal, the blood sugar levels are balanced and everything settles down until the next meal. Then the whole process begins again. It reminds me of the favorite saying used by everyone in the country of Jamaica - "No Problem".

When blood sugar levels rise up toward the top line, your pancreas must secrete insulin to try to lower blood sugar levels.

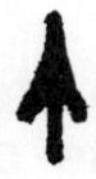

HIGH BLOOD SUGAR = **DIABETES**

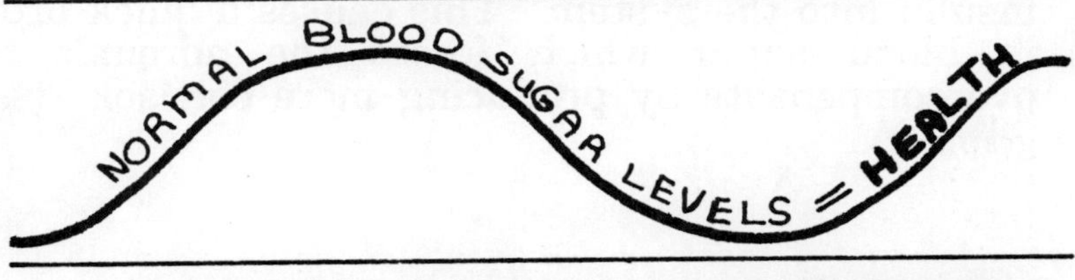

LOW BLOOD SUGAR = **HYPOGLYCEMIA**

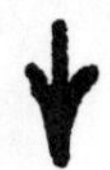

When blood sugar levels drop down toward the bottom line, your adrenal glands must work overtime to try to raise blood sugar levels.

(Graph #1)

"BIG PROBLEM"

The blood sugar balancing act usually works just fine with foods like proteins, fats and complex carbohydrates. These foods take longer to digest, so glucose is gradually released into the bloodstream over a long period of time. Problems arise; however, with simple refined carbohydrates (like sugar, molasses, syrups, white flour, etc.). These are digested very quickly and pass right into the bloodstream.

Rapidly rising blood sugar levels cause the pancreas to over-react and dump an overdose of insulin into the system. This causes a quick drop in blood sugar which forces the adrenals to overcompensate by producing more cortisol. (See graph #2)

HIGH BLOOD SUGAR = **DIABETES**

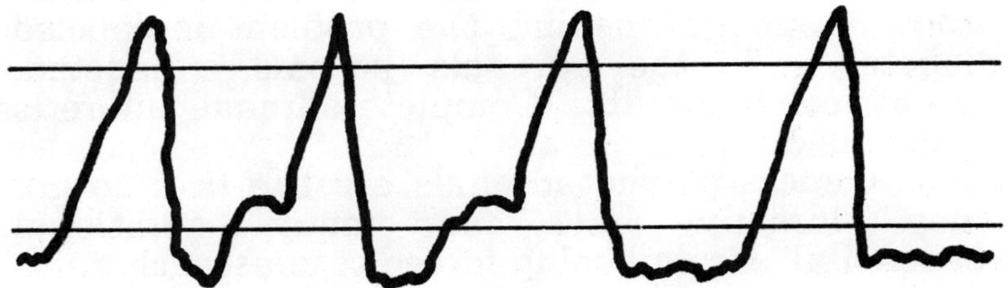

LOW BLOOD SUGAR = **HYPOGLYCEMIA**

(Graph #2)

Use of sugar, high sugar foods, and refined carbohydrates like white flour continues to cause the wild fluctuations in blood sugar levels. Each time the pancreas and the adrenals are "squeezed" to release more hormones. After being "squeezed" several times a day, everyday, for weeks, months or years, one of the glands will become exhausted and fail.

If the pancreas fails and can no longer produce enough insulin, the problem is labeled diabetes. It the adrenals become exhausted, hypoglycemia results. Complete adrenal failure is Addisons disease.

Generally, the adrenals are the first to go. They already have so many additional responsibilities and being forced to constantly raise blood sugar levels proves to be too much of a burden. Without the help of your adrenals, you're forced into a seat on the hypoglycemia roller-coaster..."Big Problem"!

Foods high in refined sugar or white flour, will cause the pancreas to produce excess insulin which drops blood sugar levels. Since your body desparately needs to raise these low blood sugar levels, you immediately get cravings for more of these type foods.

It may be something loaded with more sugar like sodas, chocolate, candy bars, or chewing gum. Things that quickly dump sugar into the blood. Or, it may be substances that "squeeze" the adrenals even harder forcing them to raise blood sugar levels. Things like cigarettes, coffee, tea, alcohol, marijuana or drugs all work by stimulating or squeezing the adrenals. As the adrenals become increasingly weaker, it takes more and more of these stimulants to work. This can lead to dependence, abuse and addiction.

Everyone seems to have their favorite "fix" to deal with hypoglycemia. Regardless of which one they use, it can only give temporary relief because all of them perpetuate the wild cycle of blood sugar fluctuation. Remember that any fast rise in blood sugar will bring on a fast drop (as long as the pancreas continues to work)! (See graph #3)

HIGH BLOOD SUGAR = **DIABETES**

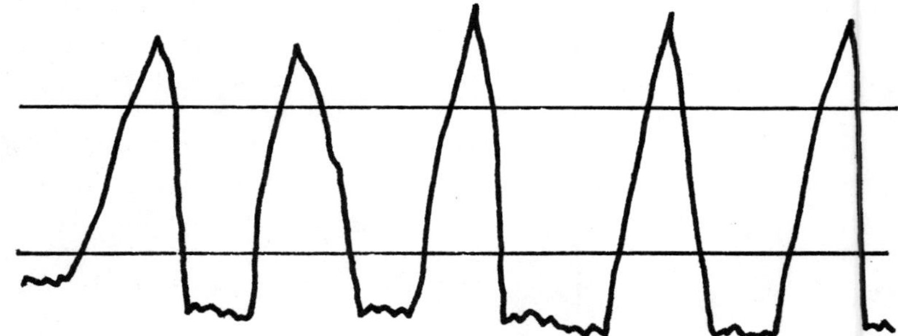

LOW BLOOD SUGAR = **HYPOGLYCEMIA**

(Graph #3)

SO WHAT?

You might be asking "what does all of this have to do with all of those questions I had to answer?" And, "even if I do eat sweets and maybe occasionally have low blood sugar...so what?"

Well besides "squeezing" your adrenals and pancreas down to the point they can no longer function, which can lead to diabetes or Addison's disease (where the adrenals stop working), you may be experiencing other problems you never thought could be connected to something as simple as sugar or white flour.

The first problem to show up involves the areas of the body that can't store glucose. When your blood sugar drops, these areas have no reserves to call on and you will experience some common symptoms. Nervous tissue (the brain, nerves, etc.), the retina of the eye and the skin can't store glucose. Because of this, hypoglycemia can be directly responsible for headaches, nervousness, shakiness, irritability, blurred vision, allergies, skin problems, etc., etc., etc. If you experience any of these when you skip a meal or go too long without a "fix" watch out!

As we cover some more specific problems related to hypoglycemia, you'll probably begin to see how every one of those questions you answered "yes" to can be a sign of low blood sugar problems.

CHAPTER 3

COMMON PROBLEMS LINKED TO HYPOGLYCEMIA

After reading this chapter it might seem like all of the world's problems could be eliminated just by correcting low blood sugar problems. You and I both know this isn't the case. There's no one solution that will correct <u>all</u> problems. At best, correcting hypoglycemia could probably solve only 95% or 98% of them.

Seriously, it is the common link to hundreds if not thousands of disease processes. I'm certain it contributes to a very large degree of the child abuse, alcoholism, drug addiction, crime, illness and family disharmony so common today.

Let's look at some of the ways hypoglycemia is linked to these problems.

Physical Impairments

Fatigue:

During low blood sugar periods, the energy needs of the body cannot always be met. This results in a feeling of constant tiredness. It brings on weakness and shaky-type tremors especially between meals or when under stress. Insomnia and the inability to go back to sleep after waking are both common problems associated with hypoglycemia. (Many suspect that waking from a sound sleep is the body's way of stimulating the adrenals in an effort to increase low blood sugar levels.)

Without proper glucose levels, you may constantly need rest. This accounts for another common characteristic of hypoglycemia: always wanting to lie down,especially when reading or watching television.

Pain:

Headaches,particularly behind the eyes or limited to one side of the head, joint aches and muscle soreness can all be caused by hypoglycemia.

The adrenal hormone cortisol,which helps to raise blood sugar levels,is also your body's natural anti-inflammatory weapon. If the supplies of this hormone are depleted in the adrenals effort to constantly stabilize blood sugar levels, inflammation problems will go unchecked. Conditions like arthritis, muscle injuries, joint disease, allergies and immune system diseases will be allowed to flourish.

Drug manufacturers have synthetically produced this marvelous hormone and I'm sure you're familiar with cortisone injections. While we're on the subject, you might want to know one of the big problems with this drug. It may temporarily relieve pain and inflammation of arthritis or allergies or other problems, but prolonged use can cause your adrenals to stop their production of cortisol (cortisone). When your adrenals detect high levels of the drug circulating in the blood stream, they halt any additional production. If levels stay high from repeated injections or oral use of the drug, the adrenals may lose their ability to produce the hormone. Repeated doses also inhibit antibody production. Without this natural defense, your immune system is weakened leaving you susceptible to disease and infection. Permanent immune system damage is not at all an uncommon side-effect of repeated cortisone injections. Additional side effects include accelerated development of high blood pressure, atherosclerosis and gastric ulcers.

If more efforts were spent in helping the adrenals to rebuild (correcting hypoglycemia, avoiding stress, etc.), and function as they should, the success in treating allergies, arthritis and other inflammatory conditions would increase dramatically..

Visual Disturbances:

If you recall, three crucial areas are unable to store extra glucose and are therefore dependent directly on blood sugar levels. They are nervous tissue, the retina of the eye and the skin.

Hypoglycemia is very often associated with blurred vision, seeing double and extreme sensitivity to light. If you feel the constant need for sunglasses or if you're bothered immensely by automobile headlights at night, it very well could be blood sugar related.

Coordination:

If you're anything like me, you need all the coordination you can get! (And sometimes it still doesn't seem like enough!) Being able to walk and move gracefully is a learned response controlled by the brain and nervous system. The brain always needs a rich blood supply carrying just the right amount of glucose and oxygen. Hypoglycemia can interrupt this supply and those hard working adrenal glands have even another responsibility in this area.

Cortisone works with another adrenal hormone called epinephrine, also called adrenaline. It's the one that enables some people to pick up cars or perform other amazing feats during stressful situations. Anyway, these two hormones work together during times of stress. Together they constrict blood vessels (causing blood pressure to increase) and they make the heart beat faster and pump more blood.

Every time you stand up, these two hormones are needed. The blood pressure must rise and the heart beat a little faster to quickly get blood up to the brain. With hypoglycemia (and hypoadrenia -- low adrenals), you will frequently experience a blackout or dizzy-type feeling especially if you stand up quickly. Lightheadedness, fainting or sinking spells and lack of coordination can all be a result of weak adrenal glands.

Circulation:

The same effects caused by cortisol and epinephrine above explains how hypoglycemia can cause heart palpitations (rapid beating), and low blood pressure which can result in poor circulation to the hands and feet.

Fluid Retention:

In addition to producing over 50 different known hormones, the adrenal glands are instrumental in regulating the amount of water in your body.

Water balance depends on the proper ratio of two minerals in the body...sodium (salt) and potassium. The inside of every cell contains potassium and it must be balanced electrically by the right amount of sodium surrounding the outside of the cell.

As you might have guessed, your adrenals, which conveniently sit right on top of each kidney, determine how much water leaves or stays in your body. They perform this miracle by telling the kidney whether to save or excrete sodium or potassium.

Before this gets too complicated, I'll just say that overworked, exhausted adrenals (from hypoglycemia) don't keep enough sodium. Instead, they keep too much potassium in the body. This explains the craving for salt and salty foods by hypoglycemics.

Remember how I said potassium is inside the cells? Well, as these overworked adrenals continue to keep more and more potassium, the inside of the cells become full of potassium. For everything to work properly, the potassium on the inside must be balanced with the sodium on the outside. Since there's not enough sodium, your body does the next best thing....it pumps water into the cell to dilute the potassium. This causes swelling in the cells and an increased need for more water in the body. While individual cells may be swollen with water, other parts of your body actually become dehydrated.

This is why hypoglycemics (with hypoadrenia) crave salt and can have problems with swollen fingers, hands, ankles, feet, etc. Many times, either the doctor or the patient will try to treat this problem with diuretics or water pills. This is the worst thing to do! It pulls more water into the cells, causing more dehydration and increased cravings for salt.

Hypoglycemia (with hypoadrenia) is one instance when a little sodium added to the diet could actually help reduce fluid retention problems. Instead of table salt, use foods high in sodium like zucchini squash, celery and green beans. Also, don't forget to drink 8 glasses of water a day!

Boy! If I haven't confused you by now, I'll stop trying. Just remember that hypoglycemia in a round-about-way can cause cravings for salt, swelling and dehydration.

I have one patient who can instantly tell when her adrenals are exhausted. Almost instantly,after drinking a glass of wine, her ankles and feet will almost double in size from the swelling. (Alcohol is one of the adrenal glands worst enemies. It is practically all refined carbohydrates which causes a rapid rise in blood sugar levels. It is one of those adrenal "squeezers" we talked about. The sound of a beer being popped open is enough to make even the strongest adrenals run for cover!)

Mental Impairment

Your brain feeds on glucose. When blood levels of glucose are low, it becomes impossible to think straight or concentrate. Forgetfulness and confusion are common.

It's not difficult to understand why so many children have difficulty in school. Many thousands are hypoglycemic.

Practically everyone at times wonders if their memory is beginning to fail. Especially with the ever-growing fear of Alzheimer's disease. The large majority of these worries could be put to rest by correcting low blood sugar problems. Retaining mental alertness and memory requires practice and effort, but it also depends on the brain being supplied with a constant non-fluctuating supply of glucose.

Mental Illness

Being unable to think clearly makes it difficult to make decisions. It brings on constant worrying and unfounded fears. It causes a feeling described as being "out of control" or "out of touch with reality". Depression, guilt, crying spells are all symptoms of hypoglycemia. Rapid personality swings follow exactly the up and down roller coaster of hypoglycemia. Suicides, nervous breakdowns and psychological problems can all result from repeated episodes of low blood sugar.

Depression (sadness combined with hopelessness) and antisocial behavior are two conditions that continue to fill our mental institutions. The hypoglycemia patient can easily pass medical and laboratory examinations with flying colors. But if he or she mentioned having even a fourth of the hypoglycemic symptoms we've covered, they would instantly be referred for psychiatric counseling.

Unfortunately, most psychiatrists don't even recognize low blood sugar as a cause of mental problems. That leaves powerful mood altering drugs and mental institutions as their choice of therapies. Institutionalized patients may become even more troublesome while they try to adjust to a diet which permits coffee, cigarettes and between meal sweets offered as rewards for good behavior.

Weakened Immune System

The adrenal glands are a vital link in your overall immune system and your ability to stay well while being exposed to thousands of bacteria, viruses and irritants everyday. Without an adequate and regulated supply of hormones like cortisol; allergies, asthma, colds, flu and practically every other ailment or disease could be life-threatening.

Breathing Problems

If you suffer from asthma, bronchitis or lung problems, there's a strong possibility that hypoglycemia and weak adrenals are involved. This is especially true if your symptoms are relieved by any of the prescription inhalers now on the market. Many contain drugs which mimic the actions of adrenal hormones like epinephrine.

Epinephrine produced by healthy adrenal glands does much more than just help cortisol constrict blood vessels. (See coordination under this section). In your bronchial tubes, it helps relax the smooth muscles that allow air to flow into the lungs. In the lungs themselves, it constricts the small blood vessels which in turn slow mucus production.

Without adequate epinephrine, the smooth muscles contract making the bronchial tubes narrower. This makes it more difficult to breath. Low levels of epinephrine also cause excess mucus formation leading to bronchitis and lung congestion. Inhalers containing epinephrine-like drugs can bring almost instant relief when their mist comes in contact with bronchial tubes and lung tissue. When you find that a short squirt from an inhaler helps, it's time to think seriously about getting to the cause of the problem...weak adrenal gland function.

You may remember a few years back, when reports began to surface claiming that new discoveries showed that asthma was brought on totally by emotional disturbances. Doctors would place asthma patients under emotional stress and this would trigger asthma attacks. It was therefore concluded that asthma was all in the patient's mind. What they failed to realize,was the adrenals were exhausted. When the patients were subjected to the extra stress, their adrenals were so weak they couldn't respond by producing the additional epinephrine needed. The bronchial tubes constricted, the mucus membranes swelled and put out more mucus which are the makings of an asthma attack. (As you'll see in the chapter on how to strengthen your adrenals, stress can play just as an important role as diet.)

If you have asthma, bronchitis, lung congestion, emphysema or any other breathing difficulties, hypoglycemia and/or hypoadrenia problems need to be corrected!

Diabetes-Hyperglycemia

It's the 3rd most common cause of death by disease in this country. About 11 million people in the U.S. have diabetes or 1 in every 20 people. Over 1 million of these are dependent on insulin injections because the pancreas has failed (Type I). The other 10 million diabetics have what is called non-insulin dependent diabetes (Type II). Out of this 10 million, over half don't even know they have the disease.

Type I diabetes occurs when the pancreas quits producing the insulin needed to lower blood sugar levels. It was thought that this type of diabetes was inherited,but it now appears that only a weakness or tendency to develop the disease is inherited. By eating the proper diet, which emphasizes complex carbohydrates, and not over working the pancreas, those born with the weakness can decrease if not totally stop development of the disease.

In Type II diabetes, the pancreas produces enough insulin but some of the insulin doesn't work properly. Much of the insulin produced is "bound up" with some antagonist that cancels it's ability to handle blood sugar. Several research studies, clinics and independent organizations like the Pritikin Research Foundation have shown time and time again that with proper diet, exercise and weight management, the pancreas can produce enough of the "unbound" insulin to enable the body to control blood sugar.

Even though diabetics can many times control the blood sugar levels with diet, exercise or even insulin, the artery damage that diabetes causes may still occur.

Around 50% of diabetics die of heart attacks. Almost 80% die from some form of blood vessel disease. Diabetes is the major cause of impotency. Its three most common complications are blindness,amputations (due to small blood vessel damage) and heart attacks. The chance of kidney damage is seven times greater for the diabetic when compared to the non-diabetic. The chances of skin and urinary tract infections is also greatly increased.

It might surprise you to learn that the diet recommended for most diabetics is exactly the one recommended for hypoglycemia. It might seem strange that the same diet could help both a high blood sugar problem and a low blood sugar problem. But if you remember, the best thing you can do to help both the adrenal glands and the pancreas is to avoid drastic blood sugar fluctuations. Sucrose (white table sugar) is said to be the main cause of diabetes with white flour following as second. Both of these products unquestionably cause drastic blood sugar fluctuations.

Heart And Blood Vessel Disease

This deadly killer stays #1 with help from both diabetes and hypoglycemia.

Diabetes causes enormous damage to blood vessels paving the way for plaque and clogging.

After eating a high sugar snack or meal, the liver converts any excess glucose into triglycerides for storage. Those triglycerides that can't be stored are released back into the bloodstream. Triglycerides are the precursors of low density lipoproteins or L.D.L's. L.D.L.'s carry cholesterol and deposit it inour arteries, leading to blockages. L.D.L. cholesterol is considered to be bad cholesterol. Sugar,along with white flour is a leading cause of obesity which places additional stress on the heart and blood vessels.

Obesity

Constant fluctuations in blood sugar levels create cravings for anything that will relieve the lows of hypoglycemia. For many,quick satisfaction is usually found in the form of sugar.

Simple sugars can provide short term, short lived energy. Fats and complex carbohydrates digest much slower and are gradually released into the bloodstream providing long term stable energy. During dieting, most people try to avoid all fats and if plenty of whole grains, vegetables and fruits aren't eaten either, then calorie-laden sweets will be used to keep them going. Then, on those occasions where willpower is thrown out the window and the dieter splurges on fatty foods, they have a strong tendency to overdo it.

Improper dieting can actually lead to further obesity by causing glandular imbalances. Exhausted adrenals subjected to the additional stress of crash or unbalanced diets can hamper their production of male and female hormones. Regardless of your sex, the adrenal glands help balance the complex hormonal system by actually producing both male and female hormones. An imbalance here can lead to a disaster. Too many female hormones can cause gyneomastia (enlarged breasts) and lack of sex drive in males. Too many male hormones lead to excess body hair (especially on the face and chest) and some male-like characteristics in females. Even worse than the cosmetic changes, exhausted adrenals rely on the thyroid for additional support. The thyroid will eventually weaken from the added workload, making it more difficult to maintain your body's proper temperature or "set point". Your thyroid helps set your thermostat so to speak. Properly set, you stay warm by burning the right amount of calories. Set too low, you burn less calories, chill easily, have constant fatigue and gain weight on even the most meager diet.

Alcoholism & Drug Addiction

Instead of using sugar as a quick fix to raise blood sugar levels, some depend on alcohol or drugs. Alcohol depletes the precious B-vitamins which are of particular importance for normal adrenal function.

As the adrenals become weaker and weaker, it takes increased amounts of alcohol at more frequent intervals to keep the blood sugar up. By drinking frequently, alcoholics temporarily succeed at raising blood sugar and many times they don't feel the need to eat. Researchers now feel this substitution of alcohol for food may prove to be the vital link in alcohol addiction.

Roger J. Williams, Ph.D. has shown that alcoholics following a diet for hypoglycemia can stop drinking or even take one drink and stop. In effect, the proper diet uses complex whole foods to treat hypoglycemia instead of alcohol. Numerous studies have demonstrated that between 95% and 100% of all alcoholics tested are hypoglycemics. Many alcoholism rehabilitation programs ultimately fail because the blood sugar problem is not properly addressed. A successful interval abstaining from alcohol can be abruptly ended when weakened adrenals are not able to respond to some stressful situation.

To combat alcohol and other drug abuse, abstinence, proper diet, nutritional supplementation and education about abuse <u>and</u> hypoglycemia must all be part of the program.

<u>Smoking</u>

Nicotine in cigarettes and other tobacco products force the adrenals to release epinephrine. This in turn causes the release of stored glucose in the liver, raises blood sugar levels and provides the "lift" associated with smoking. In effect, the smoker is unknowingly treating hypoglycemia with nicotine. This accounts for a great deal of the difficulty associated with kicking the habit.

You may be acquainted with certain individuals who only feel the need to smoke when they drink alcohol. This is almost a sure sign of a hypoglycemic with hypoadrenia. They unconsciously are treating an alcohol-induced low blood sugar level with nicotine. This can be equated with trying to put out a fire using gasoline.

As hard as it may seem, alcoholics who smoke need to give up both habits "cold turkey" when they embark on a program to stop drinking. Most will violently defend their smoking, saying they need it as a crutch, but in reality, it acts more like a chain tying them to the bottle.

A large majority of recovering alcoholics loose the urge to smoke as their adrenals begin to rebuild and strengthen.

<u>Note:</u>

I want to clear up a misconception many people have about stimulants, whether they be alcohol, drugs, tobacco, coffee, candy, soft drinks or other similar substances. Many still believe a cup of coffee <u>gives</u> them a little lift, that candy bars <u>provide</u> enough energy to get them through the afternoon or that cigarettes <u>help</u> relax them after a stressful situation. The truth of the matter is that <u>no stimulant provides or gives anything.</u> Stimulants force or "squeeze" the adrenals to release certain hormones that help bring on the desired effect. Stimulants give nothing - they force the body to do something it normally wouldn't do at the time. Abusing the body repeatedly to perform a certain function will ultimately exhaust or even destroy the glands involved.

Once a gland is exhausted or depleted it takes more and more of the stimulant to bring on the desired effect. Maybe it now takes 2 or 3 cups of coffee to get going in the morning, or two beers to feel a buzz, etc. It becomes like whipping a tired horse...you may keep it going for awhile but sooner or later you're going to be looking for a new horse.

The point to make is that no pill, drug, drink or whatever,actually contains any energy, lift, miracle or good feeling. They only work by taking advantage of certain body functions. The body is truly a miraculous creation and it can literally perform miracles. As we learn more about it maybe we'll think twice before chemically harassing it!

Crime

Several excellent studies have addressed the relationship between criminals and hypoglycemia. One particularly interesting study was performed by Alexander Schauss who at the time was Director of the County Probation Department in Pierce County, Washington.

Criminals on probation were divided into two groups. One group was required to attend classes on nutrition in addition to personal nutritional counseling sessions with their probation officers. The second group followed the normal departmental procedures with no nutritional education or dietary advice.

The subsequent arrest records of the two groups differed so greatly that Schauss made the following statement: "One of the easiest measures for preventing crime would be to eliminate all non-essential sources of sugar in the diet."

Another study in Cuyahoga Falls, Ohio by Barbara Reed, the chief probation officer of municipal court,concluded that low blood sugar is the major cause of much of the crime occurring in this country today.

In her initial study, she evaluated 106 probationers under her jurisdiction. Over 80% showed strong signs of hypoglycemia. Mrs. Reed worked with each one to set up a proper diet program. None of the individuals that followed the program had problems with the court again. The response to the program was astounding. Many of the probationer's families adopted the diet and experienced better family interaction, improvement in job performance, school work and increased stability in their home life.

Mrs. Reed commented: "Never before has the court had such a tool for working with the many ill people who find themselves in court. We wonder what the results would be if this method of treatment could be also applied to those sentenced in jail."

Mrs. Reed later reported on the study to the Senate Select Committee on Nutrition and Human Needs and was written up on the front page of the Wall Street Journal that same month (July, 1977).

Family Problems

After understanding the bazaar symptoms associated with hypoglycemia, it's not difficult to see how an entire family can be torn apart by one hypoglycemic. A hypoglycemic spouse with wild unpredictable mood swings, unreasonable fears and worries, headaches and depression who treats the problem with alcohol or drugs could break up the best of families.

To add to the confusion, normally several members of the same family are hypoglycemic...after all they do follow essentially the same diet and lifestyle.

Several hypoglycemics living under the same roof and trying to cope with today's pressures will stretch even the strongest bonds of love and patience.

Fortunately, there are some very easy steps that can be taken to help correct low blood sugar problems.

When blood sugar levels rise up toward the top line, your pancreas must secrete insulin to try to lower blood sugar levels.

HIGH BLOOD SUGAR = **DIABETES**

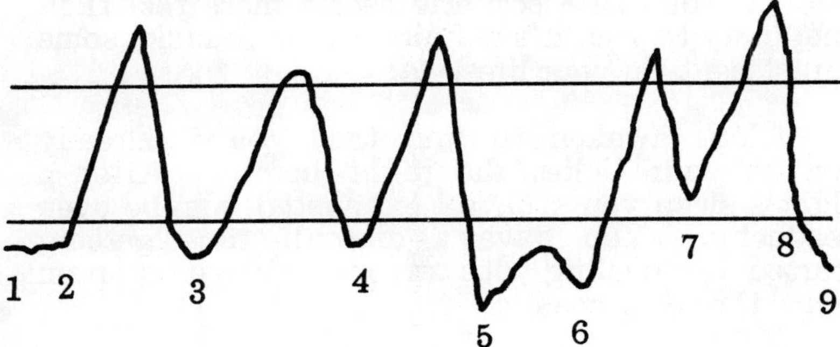

LOW BLOOD SUGAR = **HYPOGLYCEMIA**

When blood sugar levels drop down toward the bottom line, your adrenal glands must work overtime to try to raise blood sugar levels.

(Graph #4)

Obviously everybody with hypoglycemia isn't bothered by <u>all</u> of the problems we just mentioned, otherwise, half the country would either be in prison or mental institutions. Just for fun let`s take an imaginary ride on the hypoglycemia roller coaster,and get a better feeling of how most hypoglycemics live each day. (The numbers of each stage below correspond to the numbers on the accompanying blood sugar Graph #4.)

If this little scenario seems more real than imaginary to you, it's definitely time to make some adjustments in your lifestyle.

1. You awaken to find that you've already bought your ticket the night before. After a night's sleep you still feel exhausted, maybe even headachy. You have a difficult time getting started and dealing with anyone until you step on board the roller coaster.

2. That first cup of badly needed coffee, sweet roll, soda or cigarette gets both you and the coaster rolling. This shoots up your blood sugar and gets you ready for the day.

3. A hour and a half to two hours later, your ride takes a dip about mid-morning. Dragging and irritable, you go for the snack. Another cup of coffee, another soda, candy bar,etc.

4. Thank goodness it's lunch time. You're starving and starting to lose your patience. Since your dieting, lunch is limited to salad, diet soft drink and maybe a small, small dessert. Just the thing needed to set you up for another blood sugar nose dive.

5. That afternoon, your headache is back. You could take a nap if you didn't have so much to do.

Nothing seems to help. The kids are irritable and wild, the traffic is unbearable, you're starving and totally fatigued. Maybe a soda, candy bar, or some ice cream will help.

6. Didn't think you could make it to supper after an hour of self imposed silence (to keep from biting everyone's head off), you eat like it was your last meal on earth.

7. Finally you can plop down in front of the T.V. for some well-deserved rest. After a couple of hours, you feel that urge for an evening snack. A small bowl of ice cream would be good, one more piece of pie or maybe an after dinner drink; after all, you've already blown the diet at dinner.

8. The chocolate covered ice cream was good but you're so tired you can barely keep your eyes open. Maybe a good night's rest will get rid of the headache.

9. It wasn't the most enjoyable ride. The possibilities of tomorrow being better looks pretty slim since your high-sugar evening snack just bought another ticket for the same ride in the morning.

CHAPTER 4

TREATING THE PROBLEM-NOT THE SYMPTOMS

If you have a low blood sugar problem it should be obvious by now that it's not from a deficiency of sugar! In the same light, depression is not a symptom of a Valium deficiency, nor headaches caused by an aspirin deficiency or constipation caused by a laxative deficiency, etc.,etc. Each of these problems are merely symptoms of some other underlying health problem.

To enjoy good health you can't treat just the symptoms when a problem arises. Symptoms are warning signs we receive telling us that deeper problems exist. Knowing and correcting the underlying cause of health problems eliminates the symptoms allowing your body to continue its marvelous miracle of life. Chasing and covering up symptoms starts a never-ending search for quick "fixes" while ignoring underlying problems which will continue to erode your health.

Anytime you talk about hypoglycemia, you must talk about the adrenal glands. After all, hypoglycemia is low blood sugar and the adrenals raise low blood sugar levels.

We've already covered many of the various functions of these two walnut-sized glands that sit atop of each kidney, but after you learn just how hard these little rascals work, you'll see why giving them a little support will be in your best interest.

A complete failure of the adrenals, called Addison's disease, fortunately is not common. If this does happen, hormone medication is essential to preserve life. A more common occurrence is hypoadrenia -- where the glands are not quite capable of meeting all of the demands on them.

Hypoadrenia is not talked about much or diagnosed often in the medical community because it is not normally found in standard laboratory testing. Most laboratory tests are only designed to detect the complete failure of the adrenals. However, doctors familiar with the condition can easily recognize the problem from its symptoms and from the results of a good patient history and general examination. One of the screening procedures that should be a part of every physical examination involves taking the blood pressure in 3 different positions and then checking for what is called Ragland's sign. If you have a blood pressure cuff at home and know how to use it, you might want to try the test yourself.

BLOOD PRESSURE TEST FOR HYPOADRENIA (RAGLAND'S SIGN)

First have someone record your blood pressure while lying on your back, then quickly sit upright and have it taken again. Then once more standing. Normally with the help of your adrenal glands, your blood pressure will rise between 4 and 10 points (mm. of Hg.) going from the lying to standing position. If your blood pressure drops (the Ragland effect) it may be an indication of hypoadrenia. This fall in blood pressure accounts for one of hypoadrenia's most common symptoms - the dizzy or "black-out" type feeling if you stand up too quickly. The drop in blood pressure and the "black out" type sensation are so common that many doctors would argue they are normal findings. With the degree of hypoglycemia and hypoadrenia in this country, they may be common findings, but they definitely aren't normal!

The adrenals have been nicknamed the "stress glands". To strengthen your adrenals, you have to be familiar with the different kinds of stress and how your adrenals are involved with each.

In the 1920's and 1930's, research by Dr. Hans Selye showed there are basically four types of stress and that each one could have a dramatic effect on your adrenals.

Mental Stress

When most people talk about stress they are usually referring to mental stress. The death of a loved one, financial inability to pay bills, a dead-end job, or not being accepted by friends or loved ones are all good examples of this stress category. There are many methods of dealing with mental stress. Relaxation techniques, meditation, yoga, prayer, exercise and forgiveness are just a few. Everyone must discover their best method of dealing with mental stress.

A certain amount of mental stress is welcome and even beneficial for your mental health and spiritual growth, but you must be able to control your reactions toward it and balance stressful activities with relaxation. If your occupation involves mostly mental work, then you can obtain a better balance in your life by relaxing with physical activities (exercise, woodworking, sewing, etc.). By the same token, if your occupation involves physically demanding activities, you can balance this with reading or other mental activities.

Oftentimes you hear of the "fight or flight" mechanism when someone discusses stress. The classic example of "fight or flight" is the caveman walking through the jungle who comes face to face with a tiger. To survive, he has to either fight the tiger or run away. Regardless of the choice he makes, his adrenal glands help him prepare for the "fight or flight". They increase blood sugar for better muscle energy and thinking ability, increase respiration for more oxygen, increase blood pressure and heart rate to better circulate the new energy and oxygen carried to the blood, and perform a host of other duties geared toward survival.

Whether the caveman fights or runs from the tiger, his activity would cause high levels of blood to be pumped through the adrenals and they would be replenished. The situation in modern times is different.

Even though you aren't confronted with life-threatening situations everyday, mentally stressful situations can cause the same response from the adrenals . Continued stress without allowing the adrenals to replenish their reserves can lead to a multitude of problems. You can give the adrenals a chance to replenish by working to <u>control your reaction to mental stress</u> and also by providing it specific nutritional requirements as you'll see later.

<u>**Physical Stress:**</u>

Physical stress results from over working, trying to do too much in one day and not giving your body adequate rest. Rest is just as important to the body as food and water. An organized routine that provides adequate rest balanced with sufficient exercise can do wonders for the adrenal glands .

Poor posture is another problem that causes physical stress. Slumping and poor sleeping positions can both place extra stress on your lungs, heart and digestive system.

Physically demanding work or trauma to the body from recreation or sports activity can also place undue stress on the adrenals when they are practiced without restraint.

Obesity is another common problem that places enormous physical stress on the adrenals, especially since it is commonly due to a poor diet.

Chemical Stress

This type of stress is usually associated with pollution in our environment like pesticides, automobile emissions, etc. Although these are major components of chemical stress, usually your worst source is from food. Refined sugar, white flour,the thousands of preservatives, artificial flavors and colors being used, all place an enormous burden on your adrenals. Avoid refined sugars and white flour and start to minimize artificial and heavily preserved foods if you want to strengthen your adrenals.

Prescription and over-the-counter medications are forms of chemical stress. These chemicals force the body to perform some action. You'll always have to pay more than just a monetary price for any benefits they bestow.

Thermal Stress

Quick and drastic changes in temperature place an enormous burden on your body. Getting into a overheated automobile on a hot summer day and then immediately turning on the air-conditioner to blow on your face is excess thermal stress. Leaving a warm house improperly dressed for the winter cold is another example. It is best to avoid extreme changes in temperature.

Don't go overboard with this idea, though. It's beneficial to experience seasonal temperature changes. Staying under a constant temperature with central heating and air-conditioning never lets your body fully adapt to the seasons. Your body operates on a biological clock and to be in harmony with your environment, it's necessary to experience the changes from night to day and the different seasons of the year.

As you can see, strengthening and rebuilding the adrenal glands requires careful attention to several areas. Next we'll cover specific nutritional supplements and diet changes that have shown to help. Although the diet recommendations are tailored to help hypoglycemia problems, you'll find out that anything that helps hypoglycemia helps your adrenals and vise versa.

CHAPTER 5

NUTRITIONAL SUPPLEMENTATION

When it comes to nutritional supplements there are some excellent multi-vitamins on the market. However, since multi-vitamins are best used for maintenance purposes, if you have a health problem like hypoglycemia, you may have to take additional individual supplements in addition to a multi-vitamin until you have the problem under control. This is where your doctor can again come in handy in helping you decide a proper program.

It is sometimes possible to stabilize hypoglycemia with diet changes alone; however, with the addition of certain vitamins and minerals, low blood sugar problems can be alleviated much more quickly. Let's look at a few of these helpers.

B-Complex Vitamins

Practically all hypoglycemics will benefit from a good B-complex. It's possible that a good multi-vitamin will provide sufficient amounts. Usually between 50 and 100 mg of most B's are needed. B-50 and B-100 products usually work well. Always check for folic acid which should be present. (As much as 800 mcg. three times daily is not an unusual recommendation among nutritional authorities).

Choline

300 mg. - three times daily . (Certain amounts may be present in multi-vitamins and it should be present in all B-complex vitamins.)

Vitamin C

1 gram - three times daily.

GTF (Glucose Tolerance Factor)

This is one item that can be a God-send to low blood sugar sufferers. The main ingredient of GTF is the trace mineral chromium. Chromium is absolutely essential in dealing with blood sugar problems. Deficiencies are common in the U.S. even though they rarely occur in other countries. Apparently our soils are depleted and very little reaches us through our food or water supplies. To make matters worse, chromium is particularly difficult to absorb.

There are two products rich in usable chromium. One is brewer's yeast and the other is a combination formula usually sold as GTF by many different vitamin companies.

For those who can tolerate brewer's yeast well, one tablespoon taken three times daily usually provides an adequate supply of chromium along with many other necessary trace minerals.

Some hypoglycemics must start with smaller amounts (as small as 1/4 teaspoon a day) and gradually work up to the larger amounts.

GTF tablets contain chromium as their main ingredient as well as pantothenic acid (B3) and the amino acids cysteine, glycine and glutamic acid. Recommended dosages are included with each product.

Adrenal Glandular Supplements

These products which are actually made from the adrenal glands of cattle are over-the-counter non-prescription items available in most health food stores. They should be hormone free! For dosages, follow recommendations provided on the label.

CHAPTER 6

DIETARY CHANGES

The diet for blood sugar problems basically eliminates all refined carbohydrates (sugar, white flour, etc) and it stresses small protein or complex carbohydrate snacks between meals to help avoid extreme blood sugar swings throughout the day. Alcohol, nicotine, caffeine and high sugar drinks are eliminated to keep the adrenals from being over stimulated and to help give them a chance to rebuild.

Diets for both high and low blood sugar problems have changed recently. In the past, doctors recommended a diet high in protein. After realizing too much protein could actually cause adrenal and kidney problems, more emphasis has been placed on complex carbohydrates especially whole grains, vegetables, beans, etc.

A diet program consisting of around 60-80% complex carbohydrates, with 10-20% protein and 10-20% fats is generally a good mix. (Remember other diets may vary from this. This particular program is geared for working with hypoglycemia.)

Let's look at each food group separately to better understand their "pros and cons".

COMPLEX CARBOHYDRATES

Complex carbohydrates should make up about 60%-80% of the diet. Whole grains, vegetables and fruits are the best foods you can eat. The less processing they've been exposed to the better. They provide necessary vitamins, minerals and fiber. Complex carbohydrates take longer to digest and release a slow but steady flow of glucose (about two calories per minute) into the bloodstream. Your body burns carbohydrates very efficiently, in fact, it is the cleanest "burning" of the food groups. Besides providing precious energy, their by-products water and carbon dioxide are easily eliminated through the lungs and urine.

Unrefined complex carbohydrates are also your best source of bulk and fiber. Fiber has been shown to lower cholesterol and improve bowel function which lowers the risk of heart disease and colon & rectal cancer. Fiber also protects against appendicitis, diverticulosis, hemorrhoids, varicose veins and deadly phlebitis.

PROTEINS

Proteins should make up about 20% of the hypoglycemic's diet. Proteins may be the most important part of the diet. In children they are the raw materials necessary for growth. In adults they provide the materials for tissue repair. Every minute,thousands of cells are destroyed by the normal wear and tear processes of your body. Without sufficient supplies of high quality protein, rapid aging takes place, immune and blood systems deteriorate. Your susceptibility to infection and disease increases leading to frequent illness. Shortages of protein also cause fluid retention with increased strain on the heart muscle.

Until somewhat recently, many felt you couldn't get too much protein. After all protein is the only food the liver can convert to either a fat or carbohydrate when the need arises. You could live on protein alone. This explains the highly publicized high protein, low fat, low carbohydrate diets.

Unfortunately, to convert protein to fats or carbohydrates requires an enormous amount of energy besides placing additional stress on the liver and kidneys. Excess protein increases waste products like uric acid which can lead to gout. Protein can be portrayed as the ideal food but in reality,like all foods, moderation is the safest bet. Children, someone pregnant, injured, ill, overweight, or underweight might need to temporarily increase their protein intake, but generally a diet consisting of about 20% protein is recommended for hypoglycemics.

The best sources of protein are also some of the best sources of complex carbohydrates and fiber. Whole unprocessed grains, roots, nuts and vegetables are excellent sources. All of these contain the essential amino acids necessary for human health.

When you think of protein, you usually think of red meat. While a portion of meat can be included in the daily diet (1/4 lb. daily), it does have some questionable attributes. Most commercial meats like beef, poultry, pork and even some seafood are loaded with hormones and pesticide residue. Some are high in cholesterol and saturated fats.

Breeders are now aware of consumers' concerns and have brought lower fat and "range" (hormone and pesticide-free) meat products to the market. Fish and seafood farming has just recently become a big business allowing cleaner, safer fish to be marketed. Limiting red meat intake to no more than 1/4 lb. daily also helps minimize the above problems. Concentrate on lighter meats like chicken, turkey and especially deep sea varieties of fish. If fresh fish is unavailable, canned fish packed in water can be used. Limiting meats to 3 or 4 times a week could be even more beneficial in the long run. Look at meat as more of a condiment to add flavor to a particular meal, or as a side dish instead of using it as the main dish.

Other animal products are protein rich. Many however, have a high fat content and should be used in moderation. Milk products especially yogurts, uncreamed cottage cheese and the low-fat white cheeses are recommended over the higher fat products. Eggs are another good source of protein. There has been a lot of publicity about eggs being a problem if you're watching cholesterol, when in actuality, eggs aren't the problem.. Numerous studies have shown this. In fact, a recent study in the **British Medical Journal**, Volume 294, Page 333, showed that 7 eggs a week when combined with a low fat, high carbohydrate, high fiber diet did not have an effect on cholesterol levels.

Eggs do contain a high amount of cholesterol and because of this, they've received a lot of bad press. What most have overlooked is the fact that egg yolks are one of the very richest sources of choline, a component of lecithin. Choline acts like a fat and cholesterol dissolver. It keeps the cholesterol in the egg moving through the blood stream and doesn't allow it to stack up on artery walls.

Eggs are also rich in minerals, vitamins and essential amino acids. For all these reasons many nutritional authorities (including Roger J.

Williams...the discoverer of numerous vitamins) have called eggs one of the most perfect foods. (Yes for those of us who like eggs, there may really be a Santa Claus).

Enjoy an occasional egg or two (not fried in bacon grease). In the meantime, cut back on the fats and increase fiber. I guess the egg industry should consider hiring the same people who started the egg-scare campaign. They must be some of the best people in the publicity business if after 20 years, people are still afraid of eggs.

FATS

Fats are the items most abused in today's "modern" diet. Research continues to show that our high fat diets are responsible for heart attacks, arteriosclerosis, obesity, high blood pressure and even some forms of cancer. The normal American diet is 40% to 60% fat. Fats should make up about 10%-20% of the hypoglycemic diet.

Animal fat is of the very worst kind. Margarine and hard white shortening are also particularly dangerous. Even those made from vegetable oils. Although they don't contain cholesterol, the hydrogenation or hardening process chemically changes them into saturated fats. Avoid these products completely!

Occasional and limited use of butter, milk, low fat cheese is recommended over any use of margarine and hydrogenated products.

Nuts and seeds are a good source of fat. Again, moderation is the key since it doesn't take much when you're restricting fat intake to only 10%-20% of the total calories.

You shouldn't have to worry about getting enough fats in the diet. More than enough will be eaten if you include the 1/4 lb. of meat daily. (And since we're all human, those occasional indiscretions will also be a source of unnecessary fat, I'm sure.)

FREQUENCY OF MEALS

One very important aspect of using your diet to help correct blood sugar problems involves eating frequently. (If you're afraid of gaining weight, keep reading! I'll show you why this won't happen. In fact, it's an excellent way to lose those extra pounds!)

By eating as I'll outline, about every 2 1/2 hours, you can stop the blood sugar roller coaster and give yourself added energy reserves to boot. Eating three meals at the normal times and healthy snacks in between is the key.

Snacking between meals allows a smooth steady flow of glucose to enter the bloodstream. It eliminates the irritability, the cravings, the headaches, fatigue and other problems so common at 10 a.m., 4 p.m., and 8 p.m. caused by dropping blood sugar levels. Snacking can lighten the load on your adrenal glands and give them time to recuperate and perform their other duties.

With proper snacking, you won't approach every meal as though you're starved. You'll have a tendency to eat less and feel more satisfied. Proper snacking combined with nutritious meals high in complex carbohydrates has enabled thousands to reach and maintain their ideal weight. Don't equate snacking with cheating on a diet. Snacking should be thought of as one of the added benefits of eating right.

Before we look at a typical daily menu, keep in mind a couple of things. First, this is only a sample menu, you may need more or less depending on your activities, age or doctor's recommendations. Secondly, snacks are **not** complete meals. It's easy to get carried away with the snacking...don't!

TYPICAL DAILY MENU

<u>7:30 A.M. BREAKFAST</u>

One or two eggs -

Poached,soft boiled,scrambled, or even "over easy" if you use a non-stick skillet or a small amount of spray-on cooking oil. (No Frying!)

Toast or Muffin- Whole grain

Whole Orange or 1/2 Grapefruit

1/3 Baked Potato-

Cooked the night before. Can be browned or heated in the non stick skillet used above,and seasoned with salt and pepper and a small dab of yogurt.

OR

<u>**Hot Whole Grain Cereal**</u>**-**

Cooked with mixed fruit or 1/2 banana, skim milk and a dash of cinnamon.

10:00 a.m. Mid-Morning Snack

Any 1 of the following:

- Whole apple or any single piece of fruit
- Whole wheat muffin
- Small square of light colored cheese with wheat cracker
- Cup of lowfat yogurt
- Small serving (3-4 Tablespoons) cottage cheese
- Two teaspoons of one of these: Sesame, pumpkin, or sunflower seeds
- Six almonds
- Twelve peanuts (shelled)
- Two pecans
- One walnut
- 1/8 cup onion dip made from low-fat yogurt and raw vegetables like celery and carrot sticks
- 1/2 teaspoon of peanut butter and small whole grain cracker.
- 1/2 boiled egg

etc.,etc.

12:30 P.M. Lunch

Turkey Breast or Tuna Sandwich-Made on whole wheat bread.

Raw Vegetables-Carrot or celery sticks, cauliflower,broccoli, etc.

Fresh Salad-With non-sugar, lowfat dressing

OR

Potato Soup with whole wheat crackers.

3:00 P.M. Mid-Afternoon Snack

Choose one **from** the mid-morning snack list.

Or

Eat 1/4 of the sandwich from lunch

5:30 P.M. Dinner

Steamed Vegetable Combination -carrots, onions,squash, tomatoes, etc.

Brown Rice or Baked Potato-Sprinkled with a small thin slice of turkey breast (if you did not eat a meat dish at lunch),1/2 oz of graded white cheese,chopped green onions,mushrooms,etc.

Small Portion of Mixed Fruit Salad (no sugar added)

OR

Red Beans and Rice-Corn Bread

OR

Broiled fish with lemon and onions (If you didn't eat a meat dish for lunch)

Brown Rice

Steamed Asparagus (or cabbage,zucchini, spinach)

Steamed Yellow Squash

Fresh Salad or Coleslaw slaw made from shredded cabbage and low-cal,no-sugar Italian dressing

8:00 P.M. Evening Snack

Choose 1 selection from mid-morning snack list.

Again, this is only a sample diet, the possibilities are endless. Check your local library, book store or health food store for books on low-sugar, low-fat meals. Next time you shop for groceries check out the foods in the diabetic and low-fat isle for ideas. If you live alone, always cook for two and have the left-overs the next day. Make a very small extra portion of whatever you eat for lunch and use it as the mid-afternoon snack.

CHAPTER 7

A FEW MORE SUGAR-FREE TIPS

Remember that hypoglycemia is not a disease. It is a condition, a sign, a symptom, warning you that your body cannot keep up with the stress it is being subjected to. I have outlined a pretty comprehensive program for dealing with hypoglycemia and the end results can be astonishing. When you change your eating habits to deal with blood sugar problems, you'll be making major strides in helping prevent diabetes, heart disease and a host of other killers.

Most of the changes may seem small and inconsequential...they aren't! Eliminating certain foods (sugar, white flour, alcohol, etc.) while including proper snacking between meals, increasing complex carbohydrates and taking additional nutritional supplements are all essential to a successful outcome. Make the proper changes even if it seems difficult at first. The guidance and support of a nutritionally oriented doctor familiar with the treatment of hypoglycemia can help you through the rough times (surprisingly, this may only be for a week or two at most!) Once you make the decision, stick to it!

You might notice that the program I've outlined is in many ways similar to those prescribed for diabetes, cancer or heart patients. These same diets have been shown to slow the progress of these diseases and in some cases even start their reversal. Why wait until you're suffering from these problems when you have the tools to help you prevent them in the first place? Someone once said "If we would all eat like we were diabetics, diabetes would cease to exist."

If you need to make several changes in your diet, do it gradually - except for sugar. Eliminate it totally from the start. It would be far better to make the necessary changes over a six-month or a year period than to become frustrated and abandon the whole program. Just keep in mind that it's one of the easiest things you can do to improve the overall quality of your life and overall long-term health picture.

A Couple of Extra Tips

Stay out of the sugar rut. As you stay on this program for awhile, your adrenals will strengthen. If you happen to backslide and indulge in a sugar rich snack or meal, you may not experience any of the old symptoms that used to plague you. If this happens, don't mistakenly think sugar is no longer a problem!

Not having any symptoms only means your body is now strong enough to deal with the immediate crisis. Hypoglycemic patients used to return to my office after six months or a year on the program complaining that their problems had returned. Even though many claimed they hadn't changed their diet, closer questioning usually revealed they had slowly fallen back into the sugar rut. They figured if an occasional piece of pie didn't cause problems, then maybe a soft drink or two wouldn't hurt and why not drink just one cup of coffee in the morning. Everything might be fine for several months, but eventually those poor adrenal glands are exhausted again trying to keep up with the hypoglycemic roller coaster.

Sugar is hard to kick. Sugar can be a strong addiction. Some have said it is more addicting than heroin. This may sound far-fetched but look for a second at the long-term alcoholic or cigarette smoker. Both of these addictions are methods many times used in a futile attempt to correct low blood sugar. I don't have to tell you how hard it is to break either of these two habits. We all know at least one person addicted to cigarettes or alcohol.

Dropping sugar or anything used to manipulate blood sugar would be next to impossible if you forgot to include the in-between meal snacks (or the extra supplements like GTF). Getting off sugar does require discipline, but it won't take long for you to see the benefits-not only in the way you feel, but also in the way you treat those around you.

I have treated hundreds of patients with alcoholism, mental illness, learning disabilities, severe depression, obesity and a very large majority of these problems had underlying hypoglycemia as their cause. We'll probably never know how many mental patients, drug addicts, alcoholics, child abusers, spouse abusers and criminals would be living normal productive lives if their hypoglycemia was kept under control or eliminated.

BIBLOIGRAPHY

Ballentine, R.; Diet and Nutrition, A Holistic Approach; Himalayan International Institute; Honesdale, PA; 1978.

Best, Charles H. and Taylor, Norman B.; The Physiological Basics of Medical Practice; W.B. Saunders Co.; Philadelphia; 1971.

Bierman, June, and Toohey, Barbara; The Diabetic's Book; Houghton Mifflin; NY;1981.

Bland, J.; Your Health Under Seige; Stephen Greene Press; Brattleboro, VT; 1981.

Cheraskin, E., et.al; Diet and Disease; Keats; New Canaan, CT; 1968.

Colby-Morley, E.; The Reflection of Hypoglycemia and Alcoholism on Personality: Nutrition as a Mode of Treatment; J. Ortho Psych. 11 (2): 132-139; 1982.

Douglas, J.M.; Annals of Internal Medicine; January, 1975.

Drash, A.; Influence of the Level of Nutrition on Diabetes Mellitus; (In) Endocrine Aspects of Malnutrition; Gardner, L.F., and Amacher, P., Eds.; KROC Foundation Symposia #1; Santa Ynez, California; KROC Foundation; 1973.

Fouad, M.T.; Selenium and Chromium; J. Appl. Nutr. 31:14-24; 1979.

Fredericks, C.; JIAPM 1:146;1974.
______Dr. Carlton Fredericks' New and Complete Nutrition Handbook; Canoga Park, CA; 1976.

Glinsman and Mertz;Metabolism 15:510; 1966.

Goldman, J.A., and Israel, J.; Med.Sci. 10:698-701; July, 1974.

Guyton, A.C.; Textbook of Physiology; Sanders; Philadelphia; 1976.

Ibarra, J.D. Jr.; Hypoglycemia; Postgrad. Med. 51:88-93; 1972.

Kiehm, et al; Am. J. Clin. Nutr. 29:895-897; August, 1976.

Levine, Streeter, and Doisy; Metab. 17:114; 1968.

Lyle, W.H. Jr.; Hypoglycemia Diet in the Emotionally Disturbed; J.Ap.Nutr. 33:1; Spring, 1981.

Morgan, A.F.; Effects of Vitamin Deficiency on Adrenal Cortex Function; Vitamin and Hormones, 9:162-204.

Paterson, E.T.; Aspect of Hypoglycemia; J. Ortho. Psych. 11 (3): 151-55; 1982.

Reiser, S.; Physical Differences between Starches and Sugars; (In) Medical Applications of Clinical Nutrition; Ed. J. Bland; Keats; New Canaan, CT; 1983.

Salzer, H.M.; JAMA 58:12; January, 1966.

Schauss, A.G.; Orthomolecular Treatment of Criminal Offenders; Olympia, Washington; 1978.

Walczak, M.; JICAN 31 (1-2): 2-3; 1979.

Williams, R.J., and Kalita, D.K.; Hypoglycemia, The End of Your Sweet Life; (In) A Physician's Handbook on Orthomolecular Medicine; Keats; New Canaan, CT; 1977.

INDEX

NOTES

NOTES